Coconut Oil Guide for Beginners

Knowing the Nutritional Composition of Coconut Oil

By

Angus Braidy

Copyright@2024

Table of Contents

CHAPTER 1

Introduction to Coconut Oil

1.1 What is Coconut Oil?

Coconut oil, often hailed as a versatile and beneficial substance, is a type of edible oil extracted from the kernel or meat of mature coconuts harvested from the coconut palm (Cocos nucifera). It is renowned for its wide range of applications in culinary, cosmetic, and industrial fields. The oil is derived through various extraction methods, including cold-pressing or solvent extraction, resulting in different grades of coconut oil such as virgin, refined, or fractionated.

One of the distinctive features of coconut oil is its composition, primarily consisting of saturated fats, particularly medium-chain fatty acids (MCFAs) like lauric acid, caprylic acid, and capric acid. These fatty acids are believed to offer several health benefits, including potential antimicrobial and anti-inflammatory properties. Additionally, coconut oil contains small amounts of mono- and polyunsaturated fats, as well as trace amounts of vitamins and minerals.

Coconut oil is solid at room temperature due to its high saturated fat content, but it melts easily when heated, making it a convenient cooking ingredient. Its unique flavor and aroma, reminiscent of fresh coconut, contribute to its popularity in various cuisines worldwide. Furthermore, coconut oil has gained attention in recent years for its purported health benefits, ranging from supporting heart health to promoting weight management and enhancing skin and hair condition.

1.2 History of Coconut Oil

The history of coconut oil dates back thousands of years, with its origins deeply intertwined with the cultures and traditions of tropical regions where coconut palms thrive. Historically, coconut oil has been a staple in the diet and daily life of communities in regions such as Southeast Asia, the Pacific Islands, and parts of Africa, where coconuts are abundant.

Ancient texts and records from these regions provide evidence of the early use of coconut oil for various purposes, including cooking, medicinal applications, and skincare. For instance, in traditional Ayurvedic medicine practiced in the Indian subcontinent, coconut oil has been valued for its therapeutic properties and is believed to promote overall well-being.

The spread of coconut cultivation and trade routes facilitated the introduction of coconut oil to other parts of the world. During the colonial era, European explorers and traders recognized the value of coconut oil and its commercial potential. Consequently, coconut oil became a commodity of interest in international trade networks, contributing to its global dissemination and popularity.

In the modern era, the production and consumption of coconut oil have evolved significantly. Technological advancements in extraction methods, transportation, and packaging have enhanced efficiency and facilitated the widespread availability of coconut oil in various forms. Moreover, scientific research into the health effects of coconut oil has fueled its resurgence in popularity and led to its incorporation into diverse industries beyond traditional culinary and cosmetic uses. Today, coconut oil continues to be a cherished ingredient in cuisines, beauty products, and alternative therapies worldwide, while ongoing research explores its potential applications and benefits.

1.3 Importance and Uses

Coconut oil holds significant importance due to its multifaceted uses across various domains, ranging from culinary and cosmetic to industrial and therapeutic applications. Its versatility and unique composition have earned it a prominent place in households, industries, and traditional healing practices worldwide.

Culinary Uses:

1. **Cooking Oil:** Coconut oil is a popular choice for cooking and frying due to its high smoke point and stability at high temperatures. It adds a distinctive flavor to dishes and is commonly used in

Southeast Asian, Indian, and Caribbean cuisines.

2. **Baking Ingredient:** In baking, coconut oil serves as a dairy-free alternative to butter, lending moisture and richness to baked goods such as cakes, cookies, and pastries.

3. **Flavor Enhancer:** The rich aroma and flavor of coconut oil make it a desirable ingredient in savory dishes, desserts, and beverages, imparting a tropical twist to recipes.

Cosmetic and Personal Care Uses:

1. **Skin Moisturizer:** Coconut oil is valued for its emollient properties, making it a natural moisturizer for the skin. It is often used to soothe dry, rough skin and to alleviate conditions like eczema and dermatitis.

2. **Hair Care:** As a hair conditioner, coconut oil helps nourish and strengthen hair strands, reducing frizz and preventing breakage. It is commonly used in hair masks, serums, and leave-in treatments.

3. **Makeup Remover:** Coconut oil effectively removes makeup, including waterproof formulations, while also hydrating the skin and lashes.

4. **Lip Balm:** Due to its moisturizing properties and pleasant taste, coconut oil is a common ingredient in lip balms and lip care products.

Industrial and Commercial Uses:

1. **Soap and Detergent Production:** Coconut oil is a key ingredient in the manufacture of soaps, detergents, and personal care

products due to its cleansing and lathering properties.

2. **Cosmetic Formulations:** It is used in the formulation of various cosmetics such as lotions, creams, balms, and massage oils, contributing to their texture, stability, and moisturizing effects.

3. **Biofuel Production:** In recent years, coconut oil has gained attention as a potential feedstock for biodiesel production, offering a renewable and sustainable alternative to conventional fossil fuels.

Therapeutic and Medicinal Uses:

1. **Traditional Medicine:** In traditional healing systems like Ayurveda and traditional medicine in the Pacific Islands, coconut oil is used internally and topically for its purported

medicinal properties, including anti-inflammatory, antimicrobial, and digestive benefits.

2. **Oil Pulling:** An ancient oral hygiene practice, oil pulling involves swishing coconut oil in the mouth to promote oral health by reducing bacteria, plaque, and bad breath.

coconut oil's importance stems from its diverse range of uses and applications across culinary, cosmetic, industrial, and therapeutic realms. Its natural properties and versatility make it a valuable ingredient in various products and practices, contributing to its widespread popularity and enduring relevance in modern society.

CHAPTER 2

Nutritional Composition of Coconut Oil

2.1 Fatty Acid Profile

Coconut oil's fatty acid profile is distinctive and contributes to its unique properties and potential health benefits. The composition primarily consists of saturated fats, with a notable proportion of medium-chain fatty acids (MCFAs). Here's an overview of the key fatty acids found in coconut oil:

1. **Lauric Acid:** Lauric acid is the predominant fatty acid in coconut oil, comprising approximately 45-53% of its total fatty acid content. This medium-chain triglyceride (MCT) is known for its antimicrobial properties and potential health benefits,

including supporting immune function and promoting heart health.

2. **Caprylic Acid (Octanoic Acid):** Caprylic acid is another medium-chain fatty acid present in coconut oil, accounting for around 7-9% of its fatty acid composition. It is believed to have antifungal and antibacterial properties, making it potentially beneficial for gut health and immune support.

3. **Capric Acid (Decanoic Acid):** Capric acid is present in smaller quantities in coconut oil, typically comprising about 5-8% of its fatty acids. Like lauric and caprylic acids, capric acid possesses antimicrobial properties and may contribute to the overall health benefits associated with coconut oil consumption.

4. **Other Saturated Fatty Acids:** In addition to lauric, caprylic, and capric acids, coconut oil contains smaller amounts of other saturated fatty acids, including myristic acid (approximately 16-21%) and palmitic acid (approximately 7-10%). These saturated fats contribute to the solid consistency of coconut oil at room temperature.

5. **Monounsaturated and Polyunsaturated Fatty Acids:** Saturated fats predominate in coconut oil, it also contains small amounts of monounsaturated and polyunsaturated fatty acids. Oleic acid, a monounsaturated omega-9 fatty acid, is present in modest quantities, along with trace amounts of linoleic acid (an omega-6 fatty acid) and alpha-linolenic acid (an omega-3 fatty acid).

The unique composition of coconut oil, particularly its high concentration of lauric acid and other MCFAs, has sparked interest in its potential health benefits, including supporting heart health, boosting metabolism, and enhancing immune function. However, it's essential to consume coconut oil in moderation as part of a balanced diet, considering its high calorie and saturated fat content. Further research is ongoing to explore the effects of coconut oil consumption on various aspects of health and wellbeing.

2.2 Vitamin and Mineral Content

Coconut oil is primarily composed of fats, particularly saturated fatty acids, it contains only trace amounts of vitamins and minerals. Compared to other plant-based oils, coconut oil is not a significant source of essential nutrients. However, it does provide small amounts of certain vitamins and minerals. Here's an overview:

1. **Vitamin E:** Coconut oil contains trace amounts of vitamin E, primarily in the form of tocopherols. Vitamin E is a fat-soluble antioxidant that helps protect cells from oxidative damage. coconut oil's vitamin E content is relatively low compared to other oils like olive oil, it still contributes to its overall antioxidant profile.

2. **Vitamin K:** Coconut oil also contains trace amounts of vitamin K, which is involved in blood clotting and bone health. However, the concentration of vitamin K in coconut oil is minimal and not a significant dietary source of this vitamin.

3. **Iron:** Coconut oil contains trace amounts of iron, an essential mineral involved in oxygen transport, energy production, and immune function. However, the iron content in coconut oil is negligible compared to other dietary sources of iron such as meat, poultry, fish, and plant-based sources like legumes and leafy greens.

4. **Other Trace Minerals:** Coconut oil may also contain trace amounts of other minerals, including zinc, manganese, and copper, although these levels are minimal and not a significant source of these nutrients in the diet.

It's important to note that coconut oil may provide small amounts of vitamins and minerals, its primary nutritional contribution comes from its fatty acid content. The high concentration of saturated fats, particularly medium-chain triglycerides (MCTs) like lauric acid, caprylic acid, and capric acid, is what distinguishes coconut oil and makes it unique among edible oils.

When incorporating coconut oil into your diet, it's essential to consider it primarily as a source of dietary fat rather than as a significant source of vitamins and minerals. As with any dietary fat, moderation is key, and coconut oil should be consumed as part of a balanced diet to complement other nutrient-rich foods that provide essential vitamins, minerals, and antioxidants.

2.3 Other Nutrients

Coconut oil is predominantly composed of fats and contains only trace amounts of vitamins and minerals, it does offer some other bioactive compounds that contribute to its overall nutritional profile and potential health benefits.

Here are some additional nutrients found in coconut oil:

1. **Phytosterols:** Coconut oil contains small amounts of phytosterols, plant compounds with structural similarities to cholesterol. Phytosterols have been studied for their potential cholesterol-lowering effects and may contribute to the cardiovascular health benefits associated with coconut oil consumption, although more research is needed in this area.

2. **Polyphenols:** Although present in modest quantities, coconut oil contains polyphenolic compounds with antioxidant properties. These polyphenols help neutralize free radicals and reduce oxidative stress in the body, potentially contributing to the oil's overall health-promoting effects.

3. **Fatty Acid Derivatives:** Coconut oil contains various fatty acid derivatives, including monoglycerides and diglycerides. Monolaurin, a monoglyceride derived from lauric acid, has exhibited antimicrobial properties in laboratory studies and may play a role in supporting immune function.

4. **Lignans:** Lignans are phytochemicals found in coconut oil that have been studied for their potential health benefits, including antioxidant and anti-inflammatory effects. lignans are present in relatively small amounts in coconut oil, they contribute to its overall nutritional complexity.

5. **Flavor Compounds:** Coconut oil contains volatile compounds that contribute to its distinctive flavor and aroma. These flavor

compounds, such as lactones and aldehydes, are responsible for the characteristic coconut scent and taste of the oil.

These additional nutrients and bioactive compounds in coconut oil may offer some health benefits, it's important to note that they are present in relatively small quantities compared to the oil's fatty acid content. Therefore, the primary nutritional contribution of coconut oil comes from its saturated fats, particularly medium-chain triglycerides (MCTs), which have been linked to various health effects, including improved metabolism, satiety, and heart health.

When incorporating coconut oil into your diet, it's essential to do so in moderation and as part of a balanced diet that includes a variety of nutrient-rich foods. Coconut oil can be a flavorful and versatile cooking ingredient, it should complement other dietary sources of essential nutrients rather than serve as a primary source of nutrition.

CHAPTER 3

Health Benefits of Coconut Oil

3.1 Heart Health

Coconut oil has been a subject of debate regarding its impact on heart health due to its high saturated fat content. However, emerging research suggests that the unique fatty acid composition of coconut oil, particularly its high proportion of medium-chain triglycerides (MCTs), may have neutral or potentially beneficial effects on certain aspects of cardiovascular health. Here are some potential ways coconut oil may contribute to heart health:

1. **Effect on Lipid Profile:** Coconut oil is high in saturated fats, the predominant fatty acid, lauric acid, has been shown to increase

both HDL (good) cholesterol and LDL (bad) cholesterol levels in some studies. However, it's important to note that the increase in LDL cholesterol tends to be in the form of large, fluffy particles, which may be less atherogenic compared to small, dense LDL particles

3.2 Weight Management

Weight management is a multifaceted endeavor encompassing various lifestyle factors, including diet, exercise, and overall well-being. Coconut oil has garnered attention in recent years for its potential role in weight management due to its unique composition and purported effects on metabolism. Some anecdotal evidence and preliminary research suggest benefits, it's important to approach coconut oil as part of a balanced approach to weight management.

Coconut oil contains medium-chain triglycerides (MCTs), a type of fatty acid that is metabolized differently than long-chain fatty acids found in most dietary fats. MCTs are rapidly absorbed and transported to the liver, where they can be used for energy production or converted into ketones, compounds that may have appetite-suppressing effects and promote fat burning. Some studies suggest that replacing other dietary fats with coconut oil or incorporating MCT oil into the diet may modestly increase energy expenditure and promote greater feelings of fullness, potentially leading to reduced calorie intake and weight loss over time.

Coconut oil has a relatively high thermogenic effect, meaning that the body expends more energy to metabolize it compared to other fats. This increased energy expenditure, coupled with its potential effects on satiety and fat oxidation, has led some to speculate that coconut oil could be a useful tool in weight management strategies.

However, it's essential to approach these findings with caution. There is some evidence to support the potential benefits of coconut oil for weight management, much of the research is limited in scope and quality. Many studies have been conducted on animals or small human populations, and results may not be generalizable to the broader population. Additionally, coconut oil is a calorie-dense food, and consuming it in excess can contribute to weight gain if not accounted for within the context of overall calorie intake.

Coconut oil is not a magic bullet for weight loss. Sustainable weight management requires a comprehensive approach that includes balanced nutrition, regular physical activity, stress management, and adequate sleep.

Incorporating coconut oil into a well-rounded diet that prioritizes whole foods, fruits, vegetables, lean proteins, and healthy fats can be part of a healthy lifestyle but should not be relied upon as a sole strategy for weight loss.

Individual responses to coconut oil may also vary, and some people may experience digestive discomfort or other adverse effects when consuming large amounts of fat, including coconut oil. As with any dietary change, it's essential to listen to your body and consult with a healthcare professional or registered dietitian before making significant adjustments to your diet, especially if you have underlying health conditions or are taking medications.

Coconut oil may offer some potential benefits for weight management, its role should be viewed within the broader context of a balanced diet and lifestyle. More research is needed to fully understand the mechanisms underlying its effects and to establish clear guidelines for its use in weight management. As with any dietary component, moderation and individualization are key, and it's important to prioritize overall health and well-being above quick fixes or fad diets.

3.3 Skin and Hair Care

Coconut oil has been used for centuries as a natural remedy for skin and hair care due to its moisturizing and nourishing properties. Rich in fatty acids, antioxidants, and antimicrobial compounds, coconut oil offers several benefits for maintaining healthy skin and hair:

1. **Moisturization:** The emollient properties of coconut oil make it an effective moisturizer for dry skin and hair. It forms a protective barrier on the skin's surface, locking in moisture and

preventing dehydration. When applied to the hair, coconut oil helps hydrate and condition the strands, reducing frizz and improving manageability.

2. **Skin Health:** Coconut oil contains antioxidants such as vitamin E and polyphenols, which help protect the skin from damage caused by free radicals and environmental stressors. Regular application of coconut oil may help soothe irritated or inflamed skin, alleviate symptoms of conditions like eczema and dermatitis, and promote overall skin health.

3. **Hair Care:** Coconut oil is commonly used as a hair treatment to nourish and strengthen the hair shaft, reduce protein loss, and enhance shine. It can be applied as a pre-shampoo treatment, leave-in conditioner, or

styling product to improve the texture and appearance of the hair. Additionally, coconut oil has been studied for its potential to penetrate the hair shaft and protect against damage caused by grooming practices and heat styling.

4. **Antimicrobial Properties:** Lauric acid, a major component of coconut oil, exhibits antimicrobial activity against bacteria, fungi, and viruses. When applied topically, coconut oil may help combat microbial infections of the skin and scalp, including acne, dandruff, and fungal infections like athlete's foot.

Coconut oil's moisturizing, antioxidant, and antimicrobial properties make it a versatile and effective natural remedy for skin and hair care. Whether used alone or as an ingredient in skincare and haircare products, coconut oil can help nourish, hydrate, and protect the skin and hair, promoting a healthy and radiant appearance.

3.4 Immune System Support

Coconut oil has garnered interest for its potential role in supporting immune function, primarily attributed to its content of medium-chain fatty acids (MCFAs) like lauric acid. Here are some ways coconut oil may support immune system health:

1. **Antimicrobial Activity:** Lauric acid, which constitutes a significant portion of coconut oil's fatty acid profile, possesses antimicrobial properties. It can help combat various pathogens, including bacteria, viruses, and fungi, by disrupting their cell membranes and inhibiting their

growth. Consuming coconut oil regularly may help strengthen the body's defenses against microbial infections and support immune system function.

2. **Anti-inflammatory Effects:** Chronic inflammation is linked to a variety of health conditions, including autoimmune disorders and chronic diseases. Some research suggests that the MCFAs in coconut oil may exert anti-inflammatory effects by modulating immune responses and reducing inflammation in the body. By mitigating inflammation, coconut oil may help support overall immune system health and function.

3. **Antioxidant Protection:** Coconut oil contains polyphenolic compounds with antioxidant properties, which help neutralize free radicals and reduce oxidative

stress in the body. By scavenging harmful free radicals, coconut oil's antioxidants may help protect immune cells from damage and enhance their ability to combat infections and foreign invaders.

4. **Gut Health:** The antimicrobial properties of coconut oil may also benefit gut health by helping to maintain a healthy balance of gut microflora. Lauric acid has been shown to exert antifungal and antibacterial effects in the digestive tract, which may help prevent the overgrowth of harmful pathogens and promote a favorable environment for beneficial gut bacteria.

More research is needed to fully understand the mechanisms underlying coconut oil's potential immune-supporting effects, incorporating moderate amounts of coconut oil into a balanced diet may offer additional support for immune system health, particularly when combined with other immune-boosting strategies such as adequate nutrition, regular exercise, stress management, and sufficient sleep.

3.5 Potential Risks and Concerns

Coconut oil offers various potential health benefits, it's essential to be aware of potential risks and concerns associated with its consumption and use:

1. **Saturated Fat Content:** Coconut oil is high in saturated fats, particularly lauric acid, which can raise LDL (bad) cholesterol levels in some individuals. Some studies suggest that the increase in LDL cholesterol may be in the form of large, fluffy particles that are less atherogenic, individuals with existing heart conditions or high

cholesterol levels should exercise caution and moderate their intake of saturated fats, including coconut oil.

2. **Calorie Density:** Like all dietary fats, coconut oil is calorie-dense, providing 9 calories per gram. Consuming large amounts of coconut oil without considering overall calorie intake can contribute to weight gain and may hinder weight management efforts, particularly if not balanced with physical activity and a calorie-controlled diet.

3. **Potential Allergies:** Coconut allergies are relatively rare, individuals with a known allergy to coconuts should avoid consuming coconut oil or using coconut oil-based products to prevent allergic reactions.

4. **Skin Sensitivity:** Coconut oil is generally well-tolerated by most individuals, some people may experience skin sensitivity or allergic reactions when applied topically. It's advisable to perform a patch test before using coconut oil on larger areas of the skin, especially for those with sensitive skin or a history of allergies.

5. **Quality and Processing:** The quality of coconut oil can vary depending on factors such as extraction methods, processing techniques, and storage conditions. Opting for high-quality, unrefined, organic coconut oil whenever possible can help ensure that you're getting a product that retains its natural nutrients and beneficial compounds.

6. **Individual Variability:** It's essential to recognize that

individual responses to coconut oil may vary based on factors such as genetics, overall diet, lifestyle factors, and underlying health conditions. Coconut oil may offer benefits for some individuals, others may not experience the same effects or may even experience adverse reactions.

Coconut oil can be a valuable addition to a healthy diet and skincare routine, it's crucial to consume it in moderation and consider individual factors and preferences. Consulting with a healthcare professional or dermatologist can help address any specific concerns or considerations related to incorporating coconut oil into your lifestyle.

CHAPTER 4

Culinary Uses of Coconut Oil

4.1 Cooking Methods

Coconut oil is a versatile cooking oil that can be used in various culinary applications, thanks to its unique flavor, high smoke point, and stable composition. Here are some common cooking methods for using coconut oil:

1. **Sautéing and Stir-Frying:** Coconut oil's high smoke point, typically around 350°F to 400°F (175°C to 205°C), makes it well-suited for sautéing and stir-frying at medium to high heat. Its stable composition means it won't break down or produce harmful compounds when exposed to high temperatures, making it an

excellent choice for cooking vegetables, meats, seafood, and tofu.

2. **Pan-Frying and Deep-Frying:** Coconut oil's high smoke point also makes it suitable for pan-frying and deep-frying. It can be used to fry foods like chicken, fish, vegetables, and fritters, resulting in a crispy exterior and a hint of coconut flavor.

3. **Baking and Roasting:** Coconut oil can be used as a substitute for butter or other oils in baking recipes, such as cakes, cookies, muffins, and bread. Its creamy texture and subtle coconut flavor can enhance the taste and moisture of baked goods. Additionally, coconut oil can be used for roasting vegetables or nuts, adding a delicious caramelized flavor to the finished dish.

4. **Grilling and Barbecuing:**
    Coconut oil can be brushed onto
    meats, seafood, vegetables, or
    tofu before grilling or barbecuing
    to prevent sticking and add flavor.
    Its high smoke point allows it to
    withstand the heat of the grill
    without burning, its natural
    sweetness and coconut aroma can
    complement grilled dishes.

5. **Dressings and Marinades:**
    Coconut oil can be incorporated
    into salad dressings, marinades,
    and sauces to add richness and
    flavor. It pairs well with citrus,
    herbs, spices, and vinegar,
    creating delicious dressings for
    salads or marinades for meats and
    vegetables.

6. **Popcorn:** Coconut oil is a popular
    choice for popping popcorn due to
    its high smoke point and rich
    flavor. Simply melt coconut oil in
    a pot or popcorn maker, add

popcorn kernels, and cover until popped. Season with salt, nutritional yeast, or other toppings for a tasty snack.

Overall, coconut oil's versatility and ability to withstand high temperatures make it a favorite cooking oil for a wide range of culinary applications. Experimenting with coconut oil in different cooking methods can add a delightful tropical twist to your favorite dishes.

4.2 Flavor Profile

Coconut oil imparts a distinct flavor and aroma to dishes, characterized by its sweet, nutty, and tropical notes. Here's an overview of coconut oil's flavor profile:

1. **Sweetness:** Coconut oil has a natural sweetness that comes from the fresh coconut meat used in its

production. This sweetness adds a pleasant undertone to dishes, enhancing their overall flavor profile without being overly sugary.

2. **Nutty Undertones:** In addition to its sweetness, coconut oil has subtle nutty undertones that contribute to its complex flavor profile. These nutty notes are reminiscent of toasted coconut and can add depth and richness to both sweet and savory dishes.

3. **Tropical Aroma:** One of the most distinctive characteristics of coconut oil is its tropical aroma, which evokes images of sandy beaches and palm trees. The aroma is derived from the natural compounds present in coconut oil and adds an exotic touch to dishes, making them more enticing and flavorful.

4. **Mild Coconut Flavor:** Coconut oil has a pronounced coconut aroma, its flavor is relatively mild, especially when used in moderate amounts. The coconut flavor enhances the overall taste of dishes without overpowering other ingredients, making it a versatile cooking oil for various cuisines.

5. **Buttery Texture:** Coconut oil has a rich, creamy texture that melts easily at room temperature or when heated. This buttery texture adds smoothness and mouthfeel to dishes, contributing to their overall sensory appeal.

coconut oil's flavor profile is a unique combination of sweetness, nuttiness, and tropical aromas, making it a popular choice for adding depth and richness to a wide range of culinary creations. Whether used in baking, frying, sautéing, or as a flavoring agent, coconut oil can elevate the taste of dishes and transport your taste buds to a tropical paradise.

4.3 Recipes and Cooking Tips

Coconut oil's versatility makes it a fantastic ingredient in various recipes, from savory dishes to baked goods and beyond. Here are some recipes and cooking tips to help you incorporate coconut oil into your culinary creations:

1. **Coconut Curry Chicken:**

    - Ingredients: Chicken breast or thighs, coconut oil, curry powder, garlic, onion, ginger, coconut milk, vegetables (such as bell peppers, carrots, and peas), cilantro (for garnish).

- Cooking Method: Sauté
  garlic, onion, and ginger in
  coconut oil until fragrant.
  Add curry powder and
  cook until aromatic. Add
  chicken and cook until
  browned. Pour in coconut
  milk and simmer until
  chicken is cooked through.
  Add vegetables and cook
  until tender. Serve over
  rice, garnished with
  cilantro.

2. **Coconut Oil Granola:**

   - Ingredients: Rolled oats,
     coconut oil, honey or
     maple syrup, vanilla
     extract, nuts (such as
     almonds, pecans, or
     walnuts), dried fruit (such
     as raisins or cranberries),
     shredded coconut.

- Cooking Method: Mix
  melted coconut oil, honey
  or maple syrup, and vanilla
  extract in a bowl. Stir in
  rolled oats, nuts, and
  shredded coconut until
  well coated. Spread
  mixture on a baking sheet
  and bake at 325°F (160°C)
  for 20-25 minutes, stirring
  occasionally, until golden
  brown. Allow to cool, then
  mix in dried fruit. Serve
  with yogurt or milk.

3. **Coconut Oil Roasted
   Vegetables:**

   - Ingredients: Assorted
     vegetables (such as carrots,
     potatoes, cauliflower, and
     Brussels sprouts), coconut
     oil, salt, pepper, herbs
     (such as rosemary or
     thyme).

- Cooking Method: Preheat
  oven to 400°F (200°C).
  Cut vegetables into
  uniform pieces and toss
  with melted coconut oil,
  salt, pepper, and herbs.
  Spread vegetables in a
  single layer on a baking
  sheet and roast for 25-30
  minutes, or until tender and
  caramelized, stirring
  halfway through cooking.

4. **Coconut Oil Chocolate Chip Cookies:**

   - Ingredients: All-purpose
     flour, coconut oil (solid),
     brown sugar, granulated
     sugar, egg, vanilla extract,
     baking soda, salt, chocolate
     chips.

   - Cooking Method: Preheat
     oven to 350°F (175°C).
     Cream coconut oil, brown

sugar, and granulated sugar until light and fluffy. Beat in egg and vanilla extract. In a separate bowl, whisk together flour, baking soda, and salt. Gradually add dry ingredients to wet ingredients and mix until combined. Fold in chocolate chips. Drop spoonfuls of dough onto a baking sheet and bake for 10-12 minutes, or until edges are golden brown. Allow to cool before serving.

5. **Stir-Fried Coconut Shrimp:**

- Ingredients: Shrimp (peeled and deveined), coconut oil, garlic, ginger, bell peppers, snap peas, coconut aminos or soy sauce, honey, lime juice, cilantro (for garnish).

- Cooking Method: Heat coconut oil in a wok or skillet over medium-high heat. Add minced garlic and ginger and stir-fry until fragrant. Add shrimp and cook until pink and opaque. Add sliced bell peppers and snap peas and stir-fry until vegetables are crisp-tender. In a small bowl, whisk together coconut aminos, honey, and lime juice. Pour sauce over shrimp and vegetables, tossing to coat. Serve hot, garnished with chopped cilantro.

6. **Coconut Oil Popcorn:**

   - Ingredients: Popcorn kernels, coconut oil, salt, nutritional yeast (optional).

- Cooking Method: Heat coconut oil in a large pot over medium heat. Add popcorn kernels and cover with a lid. Shake the pot occasionally to prevent burning. Once the popping slows down, remove from heat and let sit for a minute. Season with salt and nutritional yeast for a savory twist.

When using coconut oil in recipes, keep in mind that it solidifies at cooler temperatures and melts at warmer temperatures. To measure coconut oil accurately, scoop it into a measuring cup and melt if necessary to achieve the desired consistency. Additionally, choose unrefined or virgin coconut oil for recipes where you want a stronger coconut flavor, and refined coconut oil for recipes where you prefer a milder taste.

CHAPTER 5

Industrial and Cosmetic Applications

5.1 Coconut Oil in Cosmetics

Coconut oil's natural moisturizing and nourishing properties make it a popular ingredient in various cosmetic products. Here are some common uses of coconut oil in cosmetics:

1. **Skin Moisturizers:** Coconut oil is a highly effective emollient, meaning it helps to soften and soothe the skin by locking in moisture. It is commonly used in body lotions, creams, and moisturizing balms to hydrate dry skin and restore its natural suppleness.

2. **Lip Balms and Lip Care
    Products:** Due to its moisturizing
    properties and pleasant taste,
    coconut oil is a common
    ingredient in lip balms, lip
    glosses, and other lip care
    products. It helps to prevent
    chapped lips and keep them soft
    and hydrated.

3. **Hair Conditioners and
    Treatments:** Coconut oil is
    renowned for its ability to nourish
    and strengthen hair. It is often
    used in hair conditioners, masks,
    and treatments to moisturize dry
    and damaged hair, reduce frizz,
    and improve overall hair health
    and shine.

4. **Makeup Removers:** Coconut
    oil's gentle yet effective cleansing
    properties make it an ideal
    ingredient in makeup removers. It
    effectively breaks down and
    removes makeup, including

waterproof formulas, leaving the skin feeling soft and hydrated.

5. **Body Scrubs and Exfoliants:** Coconut oil's texture and moisturizing properties make it an excellent base for body scrubs and exfoliants. When combined with exfoliating agents such as sugar, salt, or coffee grounds, coconut oil helps to slough away dead skin cells, leaving the skin smooth and rejuvenated.

6. **Massage Oils:** Coconut oil's smooth texture and light, pleasant scent make it a popular choice for massage oils. It provides excellent lubrication for massage therapists and helps to moisturize and nourish the skin during massage treatments.

7. **Sunscreen and After-Sun Products:** Coconut oil has natural sun-protective properties and can

be used as a base ingredient in sunscreen formulations. Additionally, it is often included in after-sun products such as soothing creams and lotions to help moisturize and calm sun-exposed skin.

8. **Anti-Aging Products:** The antioxidant properties of coconut oil, combined with its ability to moisturize and protect the skin, make it a valuable ingredient in anti-aging creams, serums, and treatments. It helps to reduce the appearance of fine lines and wrinkles and promote a youthful complexion.

coconut oil's versatility and beneficial properties make it a valuable ingredient in a wide range of cosmetic products, from skincare and haircare to makeup and beyond. Whether used alone or in combination with other natural ingredients, coconut oil helps to nourish, moisturize, and protect the skin and hair, promoting overall health and beauty.

5.2 Industrial Applications

In addition to its cosmetic uses, coconut oil finds numerous industrial applications across various sectors. Here are some common industrial uses of coconut oil:

1. **Soap and Detergent Production:** Coconut oil is a key ingredient in the manufacture of soaps, detergents, and other cleansing products. Its cleansing and lathering properties make it ideal for producing high-quality bar soaps, liquid soaps, shampoos, and laundry detergents.

2. **Candle Making:** Coconut oil is commonly used as a base ingredient in candle making due to its clean-burning properties and ability to hold fragrance well. It

produces candles with a smooth, even burn and minimal soot or smoke.

3. **Cosmetic and Personal Care Formulations:** In addition to its direct use in cosmetic products, coconut oil is used as a raw material in the formulation of various cosmetic and personal care products, including creams, lotions, serums, hair care products, and fragrances.

4. **Food Processing:** Coconut oil is widely used in the food processing industry for various purposes, including frying, baking, and flavoring. It is also used as a stabilizer, emulsifier, and texture enhancer in processed foods such as baked goods, confectionery, snacks, and dairy alternatives.

5. **Pharmaceuticals and Nutraceuticals:** Coconut oil's potential health benefits and therapeutic properties have led to its use in pharmaceutical and nutraceutical products. It is used as a carrier oil for medicinal compounds, as well as in dietary supplements, herbal remedies, and functional foods.

6. **Industrial Lubricants:** Coconut oil's lubricating properties make it suitable for use in industrial lubricants and greases. It can be used to lubricate machinery and equipment in various industries, including automotive, manufacturing, and agriculture.

7. **Biofuel Production:** Coconut oil can be converted into biodiesel through a process called transesterification. Biodiesel derived from coconut oil is a renewable and sustainable

alternative to conventional fossil fuels, offering environmental benefits such as reduced greenhouse gas emissions and decreased dependence on non-renewable resources.

8. **Textile Industry:** Coconut oil is used in the textile industry for processes such as fabric softening, dyeing, and finishing. It helps to impart softness and smoothness to textiles and can also act as a natural water repellent or moisture barrier.

Coconut oil's diverse range of industrial applications highlights its importance as a versatile and valuable raw material in various manufacturing processes. From soap making and candle production to food processing and biofuel manufacturing, coconut oil plays a vital role in numerous industries worldwide, contributing to economic growth, product innovation, and sustainability.

5.3 Other Uses

Coconut oil's versatility extends beyond culinary, cosmetic, and industrial applications. Here are some additional uses of coconut oil:

1. **Natural Remedies:** Coconut oil is utilized in traditional medicine and natural remedies for its purported health benefits. It is often used topically to soothe skin irritations, promote wound healing, and alleviate symptoms of conditions like eczema, psoriasis, and acne. Some people also consume coconut oil orally for its potential digestive, immune-boosting, and metabolism-regulating effects, although more research is needed to support these claims.

2. **Oil Pulling:** Oil pulling is an ancient Ayurvedic practice that involves swishing oil (such as

coconut oil) in the mouth for oral hygiene and detoxification. Advocates claim that oil pulling can improve oral health by reducing bacteria, plaque, and bad breath. Scientific evidence supporting these claims is limited, some studies suggest that oil pulling with coconut oil may have modest benefits for oral hygiene.

3. **Natural Lubricant:** Coconut oil's smooth texture and natural lubricating properties make it a popular choice as a personal lubricant. It can be used during intimate activities to reduce friction and discomfort, although it's essential to choose a high-quality, unrefined coconut oil and avoid using it with latex condoms, as oil-based lubricants can degrade latex and increase the risk of breakage.

4. **Wood Polish:** Coconut oil can be used as a natural alternative to commercial wood polishes and conditioners. When applied to wooden furniture, cutting boards, or utensils, coconut oil helps to moisturize and protect the wood, restoring its natural luster and shine. Simply rub a small amount of coconut oil onto the wood surface, allow it to penetrate for a few minutes, then buff away any excess with a clean cloth.

5. **Leather Conditioner:** Coconut oil can be used to condition and protect leather goods such as shoes, bags, belts, and furniture. It helps to moisturize and soften the leather, preventing it from drying out and cracking over time. Apply a small amount of coconut oil to a soft cloth and gently rub it into the leather in a circular motion. Allow the oil to penetrate the

leather, then buff away any excess with a clean cloth.

6. **Pet Care:** Coconut oil is safe for use on pets and can provide various benefits for their skin, coat, and overall health. It can be applied topically to soothe dry, itchy skin, treat minor cuts or abrasions, and promote a shiny, healthy coat. Some pet owners also add coconut oil to their pets' food as a dietary supplement to support digestion, immune function, and joint health.

7. **Homemade Products:** Coconut oil can be used as a base ingredient in homemade skincare, haircare, and cleaning products. From homemade lip balms and body scrubs to natural deodorants and household cleaners, coconut oil offers a versatile and eco-friendly alternative to commercial products that may contain

synthetic chemicals or preservatives. Experiment with different recipes and ingredients to create personalized products tailored to your needs and preferences.

coconut oil's natural properties make it a valuable and multipurpose ingredient with numerous practical uses beyond its traditional roles in cooking and cosmetics. Whether used for personal care, household tasks, or DIY projects, coconut oil offers a natural and sustainable solution for various everyday needs.

CHAPTER 6

Sustainability and Production

6.1 Coconut Oil Production Process

The production of coconut oil involves several stages, from harvesting coconuts to extracting oil. Here is an overview of the typical production process:

1. **Harvesting:** Coconut palms produce coconuts year-round in tropical regions. Mature coconuts are harvested by hand or with the help of specialized equipment. Workers climb the trees to collect ripe coconuts, which are then transported to processing facilities.

2. **Husking:** Once harvested, the outer husk of the coconut is removed to expose the hard shell beneath. This can be done manually using machetes or mechanized husking machines.

3. **Cracking:** The hard shell of the coconut is cracked open to reveal the white coconut meat inside. This can be done manually using tools or automated cracking machines.

4. **Grating or Grinding:** The coconut meat is then grated or ground into smaller pieces to facilitate oil extraction. Traditionally, this was done using hand-operated graters, but modern processing facilities often use mechanical grating or grinding machines.

5. **Drying:** The grated or ground coconut meat is dried to reduce its

moisture content and improve the efficiency of oil extraction. This can be done using sun drying or mechanical drying methods.

6. **Oil Extraction:** There are two main methods of extracting oil from dried coconut meat:

   - **Cold-Pressing:** In this method, the dried coconut meat is pressed mechanically to extract the oil without the use of heat. Cold-pressed coconut oil retains more of the natural flavor, aroma, and nutritional properties of the coconut.

   - **Expeller Pressing:** Expeller pressing involves using mechanical pressure and heat to extract oil from the coconut meat. This method may yield a higher quantity of oil, it may also result in some loss of flavor and nutrients due to the application of heat.

7. **Filtering and Refining:** The extracted coconut oil may undergo filtering to remove any impurities or solid particles. In some cases, the oil may also undergo refining processes such as bleaching and deodorizing to improve its color, odor, and shelf stability.

8. **Packaging:** The refined coconut oil is then packaged into containers such as bottles, jars, or drums for distribution and sale. Packaging may be done manually or using automated filling and sealing equipment.

The production of coconut oil involves several steps, from harvesting and processing coconuts to extracting oil and packaging the final product. The specific methods and technologies used may vary depending on factors such as the scale of production, available resources, and desired quality of the finished oil.

6.2 Environmental Impact

Coconut oil production can provide economic benefits for coconut-producing regions and communities, it also has potential environmental impacts that need to be considered:

1. **Deforestation:** The expansion of coconut plantations and agricultural practices associated with coconut oil production can lead to deforestation and habitat loss, particularly in biodiverse tropical regions. Clearing land for coconut cultivation may result in the loss of valuable ecosystems, including rainforests, mangroves, and wildlife habitats.

2. **Biodiversity Loss:** Deforestation and habitat destruction associated with coconut oil production can threaten biodiversity by reducing the availability of habitat for native plant and animal species. Loss of habitat can lead to declines in species populations and disrupt ecosystem functioning.

3. **Soil Degradation:** Intensive coconut cultivation practices, such as monocropping and the use of agrochemicals, can contribute to soil degradation and erosion. Soil erosion can lead to nutrient depletion, loss of soil fertility, and reduced agricultural productivity over time.

4. **Water Use and Pollution:** Coconut cultivation may require significant amounts of water for irrigation, particularly in dry or arid regions. Excessive water use

can lead to depletion of groundwater resources and water scarcity for local communities. Additionally, runoff from agricultural activities, including the use of fertilizers and pesticides, can pollute waterways and degrade water quality.

5. **Carbon Emissions:** The processing and transportation of coconut oil may contribute to greenhouse gas emissions, particularly if fossil fuels are used for energy. Additionally, deforestation associated with coconut cultivation can release stored carbon dioxide into the atmosphere, contributing to climate change.

Efforts to mitigate the environmental impact of coconut oil production include promoting sustainable agricultural practices, such as agroforestry and organic farming, that prioritize biodiversity conservation, soil health, and water conservation. Certification schemes such as Fair Trade and organic certification also aim to ensure that coconut oil is produced in an environmentally responsible and socially equitable manner.

Consumers can support sustainable coconut oil production by choosing products that are certified as organic, Fair Trade, or sustainably sourced. Additionally, reducing consumption of coconut oil and opting for alternative oils with lower environmental footprints can help minimize the demand for coconut oil and mitigate its environmental impact.

CHAPTER 7
Future Trends

7.1 Emerging Uses and Markets

As consumer preferences evolve and awareness of sustainability and health grows, several emerging uses and markets for coconut oil are expected to emerge in the future:

1. **Functional Foods and Beverages:** Coconut oil is increasingly being incorporated into functional foods and beverages, such as energy bars, smoothies, and plant-based dairy alternatives. As consumers seek out healthier and more natural ingredients, coconut oil's nutritional benefits and versatility make it an attractive option for

manufacturers looking to innovate in the functional food and beverage space.

2. **Plant-Based Meat and Dairy Alternatives:** With the rising popularity of plant-based diets and concerns about the environmental impact of animal agriculture, there is growing demand for plant-based meat and dairy alternatives. Coconut oil's creamy texture, mild flavor, and versatility make it a popular ingredient in plant-based cheeses, creams, and meat substitutes. As the market for plant-based products continues to expand, coconut oil is likely to play a prominent role in meeting consumer demand for delicious and sustainable alternatives to traditional animal products.

3. **Natural and Organic Skincare:** The demand for natural and

organic skincare products is on the rise as consumers become more conscious of the ingredients they put on their skin. Coconut oil's moisturizing, antioxidant, and antimicrobial properties make it a popular choice for natural skincare formulations, including moisturizers, cleansers, and serums. As the market for natural skincare continues to grow, coconut oil is expected to remain a key ingredient in a wide range of skincare products catering to eco-conscious consumers.

4. **Nutritional Supplements:** Coconut oil is increasingly being used as a nutritional supplement due to its potential health benefits and functional properties. Coconut oil supplements are available in various forms, including softgels, capsules, and liquid extracts, and are marketed

for their purported benefits for heart health, weight management, and cognitive function. As research into the health effects of coconut oil continues, the market for coconut oil supplements is expected to expand, driven by consumer interest in natural and alternative approaches to health and wellness.

5. **Green Chemistry and Bioplastics:** Coconut oil has potential applications in green chemistry and bioplastics as a renewable and biodegradable alternative to petrochemical-derived materials. Researchers are exploring the use of coconut oil-derived compounds, such as fatty acids and polyols, in the synthesis of biodegradable polymers, coatings, and packaging materials. As concerns about plastic pollution and environmental

sustainability continue to grow, coconut oil-based bioplastics could offer a promising solution for reducing the environmental impact of plastic waste.

6. **Sustainable Agriculture and Agroforestry:** Sustainable agricultural practices, such as agroforestry and organic farming, are gaining momentum as stakeholders seek to mitigate the environmental impact of conventional agriculture and promote biodiversity conservation. Coconut cultivation plays a vital role in many tropical agroforestry systems, providing food, income, and ecosystem services to local communities. As awareness of the environmental and social benefits of sustainable agriculture grows, there is increasing interest in supporting and investing in sustainable

coconut farming practices and supply chains.

The future of coconut oil is likely to be shaped by trends such as growing consumer demand for natural and sustainable products, advancements in food and cosmetic technology, and increasing awareness of the health and environmental benefits of coconut oil. By capitalizing on these emerging opportunities and addressing challenges such as sustainability and supply chain resilience, the coconut oil industry can continue to thrive and innovate in the years to come.

7.2 Ongoing Research and Innovations

Continued research and innovation in the field of coconut oil offer promising opportunities for enhancing its applications, improving its sustainability, and unlocking its full potential. Here are some ongoing areas of research and innovation related to coconut oil:

1. **Health Benefits and Nutritional Properties:** Ongoing research aims to further elucidate the health benefits and nutritional properties of coconut oil, including its effects on cardiovascular health, metabolism, and cognitive function. Clinical studies are investigating the impact of coconut oil consumption on biomarkers of health, such as cholesterol levels, inflammation, and oxidative stress, to better understand its role in disease prevention and management.

2. **Functional and Specialty Products:** Innovations in food and cosmetic technology are leading to the development of new functional and specialty

products incorporating coconut oil. Researchers are exploring novel formulations, delivery systems, and applications for coconut oil in functional foods, dietary supplements, skincare products, and pharmaceuticals, catering to diverse consumer preferences and needs.

3. **Value-Added Processing and Product Diversification:** Value-added processing techniques are being developed to extract additional bioactive compounds and functional ingredients from coconut oil, such as polyphenols, tocopherols, and phytosterols. These compounds have antioxidant, anti-inflammatory, and other health-promoting properties, and their incorporation into coconut oil products could enhance their nutritional value and health benefits.

4. **Sustainable Sourcing and Supply Chain Management:** Efforts are underway to improve the sustainability of coconut oil production through initiatives such as agroforestry, organic farming, and fair trade certification. Researchers and industry stakeholders are collaborating to develop sustainable sourcing practices, improve agricultural productivity, and enhance livelihoods for coconut farmers minimizing environmental impact and promoting biodiversity conservation.

5. **Biorefinery and Waste Utilization:** Biorefinery approaches are being explored to utilize coconut oil processing by-products, such as coconut husks, shells, and press cake, for the production of value-added

products such as biofuels, biochar, animal feed, and bio composites. By valorizing these waste streams, biorefinery processes can enhance the economic viability and environmental sustainability of coconut oil production and contribute to the development of a circular bioeconomy.

6. **Biotechnology and Genetic Improvement:** Biotechnological approaches, including genetic engineering and breeding, are being used to enhance the productivity, disease resistance, and quality traits of coconut palms. Research efforts focus on developing improved coconut varieties with desirable agronomic characteristics, such as higher oil yield, drought tolerance, and resistance to pests and diseases, to support sustainable coconut

cultivation and ensure future food and livelihood security.

7. **Carbon Sequestration and Climate Resilience:** Coconut agroforestry systems have the potential to sequester carbon and mitigate climate change providing multiple benefits, such as biodiversity conservation, soil conservation, and enhanced resilience to extreme weather events. Research is investigating the carbon sequestration potential of coconut palms and exploring agroforestry practices that optimize carbon storage and enhance climate resilience in coconut-growing regions.

Ongoing research and innovations in coconut oil production, processing, and utilization hold promise for addressing key challenges, improving product quality and sustainability, and unlocking new opportunities for value creation and market growth. By leveraging scientific advances, technological innovations, and collaborative partnerships, the coconut oil industry can continue to evolve and thrive in the face of evolving consumer preferences, market dynamics, and environmental pressures.

7.3 Challenges and Opportunities

Despite its widespread popularity and diverse applications, the coconut oil industry faces several challenges and opportunities that will shape its future trajectory:

Challenges:

1. **Sustainability and Environmental Impact:** One of the primary challenges facing the coconut oil industry is ensuring sustainability throughout the supply chain. Deforestation,

habitat loss, soil degradation, and water pollution associated with coconut cultivation can have significant environmental impacts, threatening biodiversity and ecosystem integrity. Addressing these challenges requires adopting sustainable agricultural practices, promoting agroforestry, and minimizing the use of agrochemicals.

2. **Climate Change and Weather Variability:** Coconut cultivation is vulnerable to the impacts of climate change, including extreme weather events, rising temperatures, and changes in rainfall patterns. These climate-related challenges can affect coconut yields, quality, and resilience, posing risks to livelihoods and food security in coconut-producing regions. Developing climate-smart

agricultural practices, enhancing resilience through crop diversification, and investing in adaptive measures can help mitigate the impacts of climate change on coconut farming.

3. **Pests and Diseases:** Coconut palms are susceptible to various pests and diseases, including the coconut rhinoceros beetle, lethal yellowing disease, and coconut leaf beetle, which can cause significant damage to coconut plantations and reduce yields. Managing pests and diseases effectively requires integrated pest management strategies, biosecurity measures, and research into pest-resistant coconut varieties to enhance resilience and reduce crop losses.

4. **Market Volatility and Price Fluctuations:** The coconut oil market is subject to volatility and

price fluctuations due to factors such as changes in demand, supply disruptions, and geopolitical tensions. Price volatility can affect the profitability of coconut farming and processing operations, posing challenges for smallholder farmers and coconut-dependent economies. Strengthening market transparency, diversifying income sources, and promoting value-added products can help mitigate the impacts of market fluctuations on stakeholders along the coconut value chain.

Opportunities:

1. **Health and Wellness Trends:** Growing consumer interest in health and wellness presents opportunities for the coconut oil industry to capitalize on the perceived health benefits of coconut oil, such as its medium-

chain fatty acids, antioxidant properties, and potential effects on heart health and metabolism. Positioning coconut oil as a natural, functional ingredient in food, beverages, and nutritional supplements can appeal to health-conscious consumers seeking alternatives to conventional oils and fats.

2. **Plant-Based and Sustainable Products:** The rising demand for plant-based and sustainable products offers opportunities for coconut oil to be used as a key ingredient in plant-based meats, dairy alternatives, cosmetics, and personal care products. Coconut oil's creamy texture, mild flavor, and natural properties make it well-suited for formulating vegan and eco-friendly products that cater to ethical and environmental concerns.

3. **Innovation and Value-Added Processing:** Continued innovation in processing technologies and value-added products can create opportunities for the coconut oil industry to diversify its product portfolio and capture new market segments. Developing specialty products such as virgin coconut oil, organic coconut oil, and value-added coconut derivatives can differentiate brands and command premium prices in the market.

4. **Sustainable Certification and Traceability:** Embracing sustainable certification schemes, such as Fair Trade, organic, and Rainforest Alliance, can enhance the marketability of coconut oil products and appeal to consumers seeking ethically sourced and environmentally responsible options. Implementing traceability

systems and transparency
measures can provide assurance to
consumers about the origins,
production methods, and social
and environmental impacts of
coconut oil.

5. **Research and Development:**
   Investing in research and
   development initiatives can drive
   innovation, improve agronomic
   practices, and address key
   challenges facing the coconut oil
   industry, such as pests, diseases,
   climate resilience, and value
   addition. Collaborative research
   partnerships between
   governments, academia, and
   industry stakeholders can
   accelerate scientific advancements
   and knowledge sharing to support
   the sustainable growth of the
   coconut sector.

Addressing these challenges and
capitalizing on emerging opportunities,

the coconut oil industry can navigate the evolving landscape of consumer preferences, market dynamics, and sustainability imperatives to build a more resilient, inclusive, and sustainable future for coconut farming and processing communities worldwide.